EATING HEALTHY ON A BUDGET

A How-To Guide

By

Duc Vuong, M.D.

Copyright © 2016

www.UltimateGastricSleeve.com

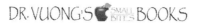

DR. VUONG'S SMALL BITES BOOKS

This edition published by HappyStance Publishing

Print ISBN-13: 978-0692778968

Print ISBN-10: 0692778969

Cover design and interior layout by Tony Loton of LOTONtech Limited.

*

Dr. Vuong's Small Bites Books provide easily-digestible pieces of potentially life-changing information. You can find the entire series on Amazon.com.

For My Patients,

who inspire me every day with their courage.

Introduction

It is health that is real wealth, and not pieces of gold or silver
– Mahatma Gandhi

Eating healthy is a constant challenge. Especially when you are working on a tight budget. It is a constant balancing act between your health and your budget. More often than not, the budget will win.

However, 'cheap' food is not really cheap. The high sodium levels used to preserve those hot dogs and pre-packaged dinners raise your blood pressure. Enriched white flour and sugar send your blood sugar on a roller coaster ride. Sodas and Tang hide empty calories that creep into your waistline. Over time these bad food choices impact your health and your medical bills. In the long run, you spend more to fix your health than you would have to maintain it.

This does not mean that you need to pay an arm and a leg for healthy food. With planning and a little research, you can attain groceries for a fraction of their retail price. You can even attain organic foods for *pennies on the dollar* if you know where to look.

This book explains how you can bring home fresh, healthy foods and drive down your grocery bill. Most of it will cover our biggest battle fields: Our homes and our grocery stores. However, I'll also go over some hidden savings in your community that you can capitalize on.

Your health is the single most important asset you have, but you do not need to break the bank to maintain it. In fact, the right planning and a little effort can even save you money!

Table of Contents

Chapter 1: Planning

*A goal without a plan, is just a wish. – **Antoine de Saint-Exupery***

Wanting to spend less money on healthy groceries is not enough.

Before you step into a store, **you need a plan of action.** Not just a spending limit and an idea of the necessary items. You need a full out strategy. The better your strategy, the more you will save.

A plan is a guide. It gives you more control over what goes in the cart and out of your bank account. A plan protects you from impulse purchases and poor choices. Most importantly, a plan helps you get the best value in the smallest amount of time.

When you first begin planning, it will take a considerable amount of time. You are building a whole new method of shopping, so this is normal. You will find ways to streamline your process as you build the foundation of your personal shopping plan.

In this book, we are assuming that you already know what you can spend in groceries for the month. Let's go over the five steps to setting your boundaries:

First: Attain your supplies

First, you will need a small storage box. This could be anything from a large shoe box to a sliding drawer from Wal-Mart. The only criterium is you want it to be large enough to store your physical planning materials: files, newspaper circulars, notebooks, calculator, etc. This will save you time and a headache by keeping your materials together and uncluttered. You will also need:

- Notebooks or an organization app like Evernote

- A simple calculator or calculator app

- A planner/calendar with ample space for personal notes. If you do not like physical planners, there are free apps that will sent you automatic alerts, such as Google Calendars.

Second: Invest in Weekly Circulars

Circulars are important to budgeting. They list out the produce and fresh meats they have on sale, along with other specialty foods, laundry detergents, and other necessities. These items are put on sale as loss leaders. They are incentives (bait) to tempt you into the store. If you are careful about your spending choices, these loss leaders can save you hundreds of dollars in groceries every month.

More importantly, if you watch over the circulars you will notice *patterns* in the sales. You'll see that Store A always puts milk on sale the week after Store B. You will see that particular food prices rise and fall in a set pattern. You will see deep discounts on fresh fruit on a particular week of the month. **These patterns will help you plan and anticipate the times you can get the best prices.**

A New Mexico Mom discovered her local store always puts free-range chicken on a buy one-get one free sale on the last week of the month. Now she always keeps money set to the side in an envelope for that week. She then buys and freezes enough chicken to last her family until the next sale. Using this method, she saves 50% on chicken simply by waiting for the right time to stock up.

Your local newspapers have caught onto the coupon and sales culture. If you do not get the local paper already, check with them about a Sunday paper only subscription.

Also write down stores you shop at frequently. Grocery stores, convenience stores, restaurants, etc. Google the store name and 'weekly circular' to find their online, download, and bookmark it. If they have an online newsletter/ email update, sign up for it to catch their exclusive deals.

Thrifty Tip: Some people create a second email account specifically for their store spam, and they only refer to it when they are planning a shopping trip. This reduces clutter in your main email account, *and* it reduces your daily exposure to impulse sales.

Step 3: Learn Store Policies

Each store has its own sales policy. The policy is almost always listed on the website. If you have trouble finding it, you can call customer service and request that they email the policy to you.

Their policy will cover very important data: Do they price match their competitors if you bring in an ad? Do they double or triple coupon values on a certain day of the week? Can you stack the store coupon and a manufacturer's coupon on the same item? This knowledge can lead to BIG savings in your planning process.

> **Thrifty Tip**: Many coupon-strategy sites provide store policy downloads of the most popular grocery chains. Some also provide weekly planners to stack sales and coupons.

Step 4: Plan a Menu

Now that you have an idea where the healthy bargains are for the week, you can pick your store(s) and plan a menu based on their sales. Don't forget to account for any special events in the coming week, like birthday parties or a school game. **You can find a basic menu planner in Appendix 1 of the book to get you started.**

If you are new to cooking, there are a host of recipes online that are perfect for beginners. You can search by ingredients for recipes on sites like Yummly and Allrecipes. Start off by bookmarking five of your favorites for dinner. Write down the ingredients onto your list. If you know a healthier alternative (whole grain flour instead of enriched white for instance), write down the alternative instead.

If you can cut out meats, all the better. Meat is expensive, especially properly raised and hormone free meats. You can drop your grocery bill drastically by sticking to other sources of protein and amino acids like beans, tofu, and quinoa. Fish and seafood is often cheaper if you live near the ocean.

If you are not ready for a meat-free lifestyle, try to stick with what is on sale whenever a healthy option is presented. There are also local options to find cheaper healthy meats and produce. We will go over those later in the book.

Cut out any junk food from your list. **Junk food is very expensive per unit.** Let me repeat so you really understand this point. Junk food is very expensive for what you are getting nutritionally. It is heavy in calories, fats, sodium, preservatives, and sugar. Worse, junk food offers very little nutritional value. Use the money saved to bring in nuts, fruits, and other healthy treats.

Step 5: List ingredients

Now that you have a menu planned, list out the ingredients you need. If you have a price, write it down. Compare the estimated total to your max budget for the week. Is there anything that can be omitted? Do you need to change a menu item or substitute an ingredient?

Once the list fits your budget, go through your fridge and pantry to see what you have. **Cross off everything you do not need to buy.**

After you have narrowed down your master list, check through the circulars and group them by store (and their final price if you know it.)

To speed up your grocery trip, organize each store's list by grouping items together by their aisle or department.

Thrifty Tip: Short on time? Take the circulars with you to Wal-Mart. They will match their competitor's sale price, and you can still use your manufacturer's coupons. If in doubt (ex: sale per pound on produce or meat) check their policy or call customer service before you go.

Now you are ready! You know what you plan to buy and where you plan to buy it. Over time, you will start to notice patterns in sales and prices. This alone will save you a lot of money. Doing absolutely nothing else, you can replace a chunk of your shopping cart with healthier alternatives. Better yet, you will not need to pay more to do it!

This is good, but we can do even better. Next let's go over where you can save money when you are shopping.

Chapter 2: Where to Shop

It's the old real estate Mantra:
Location, Location, Location. – ***Tim Carter***

You have a vast variety of *places* to shop. Not just a series of grocery store chains. In fact, you can save a considerable amount of money simply by knowing where to shop.

Produce Market

This store type is similar to a super market, but they have a much larger selection of local food, bulk grains, etc. They also tend to have fewer processed food choices.

Produce markets keep a combination of national brands and local farm products. These local products can be cheaper and fresher when they are in season.

"This summer, our local Sprouts store had a great sale on local watermelons. Only a dollar for every five pounds of melon. We got a month worth of melon for only a few dollars." – Mary J., Scottsdale, Az

Dollar Stores:

Most dollar stores are not very efficient on fresh foods. However, they often have electronics, toothpaste, detergent, spices, and other items at a lower price. Dollar Trees and 99 cent stores are hit and miss on organic foods, but many of their stores do stock unprocessed meat and produce nowadays.

Even if you do not buy food at the dollar brand stores, you can save on hygiene and cleaning products. **The money saved on household items could then go to fresh groceries.**

Farmers Markets:

You cannot get much fresher than veggies bought at the farmer's market. In addition, you can acquire other goods like honey, eggs, dehydrated meats, homemade cheeses, fresh juice, and other household goods like soap. Prices are usually cheaper or equal to organic foods in the store. Bartering or negotiating is always a fun and accepted practice.

Also, these foods did not travel for a week in a truck. They were made locally, and in most cases they have better flavor than store bought. More importantly, you will know that you supported your local community without breaking your budget.

Butcher/ Fishmonger

The most expensive thing in your grocery list is almost always meat. The butcher and fishmonger in your area import meats as needed, but they mostly deal with local farms and ranches. These are the places that you can find many local meats and fish at a good price.

In addition, you can customize your purchase. You can pick the thickness of the steaks. You can have the fat trimmed and the fish filleted. You can have them slice meat into portion sizes and slices. You can even have the meat ground without extra fat added in. Often for no additional cost.

Community Supported Agriculture (CSA)

Community Supported Agriculture is a very interesting business model. You pay a fee for a set period of time (often every two weeks for x months). **Your money helps support the maintenance costs of the farm. In return, you get a share of the harvest during that harvest time.**

You usually get 10-20+ pounds of fresh, pesticide-free produce. The farm may also add in meats, eggs, milk, or honey at their own discretion.

> **Thrifty Tip:** It never hurts to ask if they take volunteers. Some CSA's let people volunteer manual labor around the farm. Depending on the location, the work could be tax deductable. You may even receive some fresh foods for your time. If not, the exercise and sunlight would be good for you and your family.

There is a small risk involved in a CSA. Your reward is only as good as the harvest. If they have a bad year, you may get a very scant reward for your investment. On the other hand, in an exceptionally good harvest you could end up with more food than you can possibly use! This surplus will last a good while if properly frozen.

Food Depots

Restaurants do not run to Wal-Mart for their ingredients. If they are not a contract-bound franchise, they get their materials from a food depot. These places sell fresh and organic veggies, fruits, meats, and other goods in large bulk. You can find tomatoes sold by the tray, lettuce by the box, etc. In most cases, each unit of food costs a fraction of the chain store price.

The best way to use a food depot is to team up with a group of shoppers. Each person puts in x dollars (collected up front). Then a member of the team goes shopping for agreed items. Everyone who contributes gets an equal share of these deeply discounted bulk goods.

Online Stores

If you are limited in your local choices, you can still save on traveling expenses. Online stores like Thrive Market offer healthy, unprocessed foods for a fairly reasonable price.

Also, some store chains will deliver to your door if you live within so many miles of their location. Just keep track of the extra costs. You do not want your gas savings eaten up in the delivery fee.

Some local farms will also deliver fresh produce to your doorstep at a very reasonable price.

Now we have a plan, and we know where to shop. Now let's go over how to shop.

Chapter 3: Grocery Store

I can spend hours in a grocery store.
I get so excited when I see food, I go crazy. – **Cameron Diaz**

The grocery store is now our most common method of attaining food, and the stores know it. They are also aware that you live in a rushed, chaotic world where you often make split second impulsive decisions.

They know you do not always eat before you go shopping. They know what colors and cartoon characters will send children into a frenzy of desire. They know which items you will run into the store for 'just a few minutes' to get. They know what colors draw your eyes, and where your eyes will land first on an aisle.

In other words, they know how to make you buy more. Not out of any maliciousness. They are a business. They have to build their bottom line each day to stay open. However, giving into the expertly crafted temptations is not good for your budget.

In Chapter 1, you created a list. If you stick to the list, this will help you stay on budget. But what else can we do to lower the budget further?

➢ **Stick to the List:** The store already listed all its loss leaders in the circular. You spent time designing a special menu for a week, so you do not need to look for extra meal ideas. Take your list and stick to it.

➢ **Take a Calculator**: Keep a running tally of your grocery costs to make sure you know how much you are spending.

➢ **Take Advantage of your Store Card**: Many stores have a loyalty card where they track and study customer's spending habits. As a thank you for this insight, they give you special discounts, points or coupons for your use. Don't forget to use any extra savings you have to your advantage.

➢ **Grab a Hand Basket**: In "How to Cut Your Grocery Bills in Half," the authors explain how they keep a hand basket in their cart. If they grab something not on the list, they put it in the basket. When it is time to check out, they have a better visual of the extras they picked up. Most of it is usually returned to the shelves.

➢ **Never Go Hungry:** This is the scout motto for smart shopping. Hunger makes food more appealing. You are more likely to make impulse purchases, such as packages of deli fried chicken and ready made snacks. The best defense is to eat something before you go in. Even snacking on a handful of nuts or some fruit is better than an empty stomach.

➢ **Go When Kids Are Occupied:** Leave the kids with a sitter, let them stay at nana's house, shop while they are at school… however you can manage to do it. First, this removes a huge distraction. You will not be divided between your mission and childcare. You can focus solely on getting what is on your list and get out of there.

Second, fewer impulse buys will land in your shopping cart. It is easier to keep candy bars and overpriced sugary cereals out of the cart when the kids are not there. Plus kids need to be fed and hydrated. They get tired and irritable more easily. By the time you get out of the store, you may find $50+ in impulse buys, bribes for good behavior, and a pre-cooked meal tacked onto your final bill. If you do this 2-3 times a month, those extras really add up!

➢ **Know when the Truck Comes in**: To find the freshest produce possible, go in after their truck makes its delivery. Ask employees when they get shipments of fresh produce and seafood.

➢ **Shop the Perimeter First:** Fresh produce, meats, and dairy are all located around the perimeter. You will also find many loss-leaders from the circulars and stands of 'last chance" sales. The aisles have a much higher concentration of "processed foods" full of sodium and preservatives, and artificial ingredients.

➢ **Shop the Frozen Section Second**: Most people save this spot for last, so that they have the maximum time possible to get their food home. However, this is also the time you are tired and ready to check out. You are less likely to slip in extra ice-cream or extra frozen dinners if it is near the start of the trip.

➢ **Put Your Cart On A Timer.** The longer you linger in the store, the more impulse purchases you are likely to make. Get in and get out as fast as possible. This invisible clock encourages you to stick to the list and get into the checkout line.

➢ **NEVER Buy At The Checkout Line**: Forgot batteries or some razors? Go to the aisle to get it, not the checkout line. The items at the checkout counter take full advantage of your rushed forgetfulness. Need proof? Look at the 20 oz juice and water. They are nearly the same price as a 2-liter or gallon sized jug!

➢ **No Brand Loyalty:** Be loyal to the health of a food, not the name. There are many foods that are the same regardless of brand. You can save up to 50% simply swapping to a cheaper identical *nutrition label*.

➢ **Try Generics and Store Brands**: Some generics are terrible. Some are far better than their brand version. Some are completely identical to the brand, but they piggyback off the brand name's advertising and reputation. For example, they will say "Compare to [insert brand product here]."

Check the nutrition labels and try out any promising looking cheaper substitutes. It's a great way to save without a coupon.

➢ **Check The Unit Price**: Are you really getting a bargain on that fillet or bag of grapes? Check the unit price, and compare it to its alternatives. Will you get more bang for your buck out of a pound of steak or a pound of turkey? Is it cheaper to buy three pounds of apples, or a bag of apples? How much per ounce is one container of yogurt over another?

➢ **Buy Whole Foods**: A block of cheese is cheaper than shredded cheese, and it can be grated, sliced or diced as needed. Brown rice and oats are cheaper in bulk than small serving packets. A whole chicken is much cheaper than its individually packaged parts.

➢ **Consider Cheaper Cuts Of Meat**: The cheapest cuts of meat are great for burritos, casseroles, stews, and other foods. These foods also make great leftovers. Just warm them up and you have another meal.

➢ **Chicken and Turkey**: Chicken and turkey are usually cheaper than beef, and they can easily substitute the cow in any recipe.

➢ **Replace meats with other Proteins**: If you can cut meat out altogether, great! It is very possible for someone to live vegetarian nowadays as long as they are mindful of their vitamins and amino acids. Even if it is just 1-2 times a week, less meat means bigger savings. You can look to things like lentils, beans, tofu, eggs, fish, and the 'perfect protein' quinoa. Quinoa is particularly good for you because it contains all the amino acids your body needs, without the saturated fat meat has.

➢ **Avoid Junk Food**: Junk food is expensive and inefficient. It offers very little nutrition in exchange for their high fat, calorie, and sugar content. In a later chapter, we'll go over how to make your own cheaper and healthier chips and other treats.

➢ **Cut out Soda and Store Juice**: These are mostly sugar, sodium, and concentrates. This doesn't include the dyes, artificial flavors and preservatives. Water with a lemon or slice of orange in it will provide more nourishment on fewer calories. You can find lots of home made teas and fruit infused water ideas online. They will cost you a fraction of the cost of Junk Drinks.

➢ **Stock Up On Sales**: If you have been using the sales circulars to plan your trip, you already know to expect them. Stocking up while prices are low helps keep the pantry full for less. Just make sure you do not buy more than you will use or trade away before they expire.

➢ **Make Your Own Lunch Snacks**: Buy pretzels, blocks of cheese, baby carrots, etc. when they are on sale. Buy them in bulk, then separate them into baggies at home. Now you have fresh snacks at a fraction of the price.

➢ **Stock Up On Produce In Season**: When produce is in season, stores slash their prices. When the prices hit a low-mark, buy them in bulk. Freeze, jelly, or can the extra to make them last the year.

➢ **Keep The Staples On Hand**: Make sure your pantry is loaded with the staples. They keep for a long time in an airtight container. Plus they are used in a variety of healthy, inexpensive dishes. Pay special attention to oats, brown rice, millet, barley, beans of all sorts, couscous, quinoa, lentils, and dried nuts/berries.

➢ **Watch The Register Scanner**: Stores try to keep their prices accurate. However, thousands of products and constant price changes cause mistakes. LOTS of mistakes. Make sure your sale items ring up accurately. Double check to make sure you got all your discounts and coupons before ringing out. At the very least, check the receipt for discrepancies before you leave.

The savings do not stop at the store. There are lots of things we can do at home. In the following chapters, we will start to cover useful tools, tips for the kitchen, and even some interesting ways the community can save your budget.

Chapter 4: Thrifty Tools

Good kitchen equipment is expensive, but most tools will last a lifetime and will pay for themselves over and over again. – **Delia Smith**

You can make many healthier, preservative free foods on your own by buying the appropriate tools. Admittedly, there is an upfront investment. However, these tools will help you create healthy foods for a fraction of what they cost in the store.

Food Processor

A food processor helps a great deal with making various foods. You can reach a much finer consistency than you can with a blender. You can use it to mix your own whole grain pasta dough. You can grind whole grains into flour (and add nuts or berries for extra flavor and nutrition). You can make fresh salsa or puree stock for soup. You can even find directions online on how to make your own lean ground meat, no added fats necessary.

> **Thrifty Tip**: You can make your own organic peanut butter by putting unsalted peanuts and a tablespoon of sunflower oil in a food processor. Blend until it is the desired consistency. You can also add other ingredients like unsweetened dark chocolate or a spoonful of raw honey to make your own specialty peanut butter.

Juicer

Most juices on the store shelf are not really juice. They are made with imitation flavors or fruit concentrate. Even "100% juice" has a certain amount of concentrate to it, plus sweeteners, chemicals to keep it vibrant, and other additives. Look for fruit, leafy greens and berries in bulk for a great price. Look for overripe fruits and vegetables that are marked down for extra savings. You can use the juicer to make true 100% juice for your family to enjoy.

> **Thrifty Tip**: Find recipes that use the leftover rinds and pulp from the juicer. Residual pulp can be used in muffins. They often make good jams and cobblers. Even orange peels can be turned into zest.

Slow Cooker

Don't have time to cook? You can still provide delicious and healthy meals for your family.

Slow cookers are just as their name implies. They cook the food over low electric heat. Low enough that you do not need to monitor it like you would the oven. You can get house work done, run an errand, or take the free time to catch up on a hobby.

You can even throw a chicken and chopped veggies in it before you take the kids to school, and you'll have a meal waiting for you when you get home from work.

Afraid it will be mushy? Most modern models come with a timer. You can set it to start cooking automatically later in the day. There are a host of healthy recipes you can set and walk away from, even low-carb vegetarian pizza! Check out Lisa Kozich's site crockmoms.com

> **Thrifty Tip**: Slow cookers do not heat up your house like the oven does. This is especially helpful to your summer cooling bill!

Air-tight Storage Containers

If you buy cereal, whole grains, pastas, dry beans, etc. in bulk, make sure you have an appropriate vessel to store them in. An air-tight jar or dispenser will help keep the item fresh and pest free longer. Make sure they are clear so that you can see what is being stored at a glance.

Vacuum Sealer

Meat can last 4 to 6 weeks in the Styrofoam and shrink wrap packaging from the meat department. Then you start to deal with drying and freezer burn. Wasted food is wasted money.

Fresh vacuum sealed meat lasts for over a year in the freezer! If you find an amazing deal on meat or fish, you can stock up for months in advance if you vacuum seal meal-sized portions when you get home.

Deep Freeze

Bread, grains, meat, and most produce will stay fresh much longer if they are frozen. However, there is only so much space to go around. If space allows, invest in a deep freezer. This will give you the space you need to stock up when you find a great deal.

> **Thrifty Tip**: Buy your bread from the last chance rack or hunt down a discount bread store. These brink of expiring breads will keep in the freezer for up to a month without losing its flavor. However, keep in mind that all store-shelf bread is loaded with sodium to keep it fresh longer. Don't go overboard on the sandwiches in your menu.

When shopping around, make sure to check the product reviews and the Consumer Report Guide before making a purchase. For more savings, check eBates.com for rebate options. Also consider using any points rewards cards you have (Pay the balance before the day is out. That way you get the rewards without accruing interest charges.)

Chapter 5: Cheaper At Home

*You don't have to cook fancy or complicated masterpieces- Just good food from fresh ingredients. – **Julia Child***

There are many things we can do in the comfort of our home. No one thing is a 'magic bullet' to drop your grocery bill. However, together, they add up to big savings.

➢ **Cook At Home**: Recipes and cooking techniques used to be passed down in the family. Nowadays it is often seen as daunting. Especially with the huge assortment of microwave dinners and fast food on hand. You will eat healthier for less if you make these foods on your own. There are a host of free recipes all over the net, and you can sample cookbooks at the library. Get a feel for what you like to cook. You'll eat healthier, tastier, *and* cheaper!

➢ **Pack Your Own Lunches**: Those pre-made sandwiches are $4 - $6 for ONE sandwich cut in half. You can make your own lunches for less than half the cost. You can also invest in a thermos or small travel containers to transport leftover spaghetti, soups, deluxe salads, and more.

➢ **Make Your Own Nut Butter**: Put raw nuts through a food processor with a spoonful of coconut or sunflower oil. You can also add in honey, dark cocoa, dried berries, and other things to make your own gourmet butter.

➢ **Make Your Own Apple Sauce:** Remove the skin, core and seeds, then puree the apple slices in a food processor. That is all there is to it. Try out specialty flavors by adding in bananas, strawberries, blueberries, mango, cinnamon, or a spoonful of local honey. Avoid refined white sugar as a sweetener.

➢ **Know Your Meat**: Meat can stay in the freezer for up to 3 months. You can extend its lifespan to over a year if you vacuum seal it.

➢ **Freeze Leftover Soup**: A big pot of soup can last several meals. Soup will keep in the Freezer for 2-3 months in an airtight container. You can portion it for individual meals or family dinners.

➢ **Most Veggies Freeze Well**: First you want cut them into pieces. Add them to boiling water for 2-3 minutes. Then drain off and dry. This process, known as blanching, prepares the pieces for several months in the freezer.

To make them easier to manage, spread them in a single layer on wax paper. Then freeze them for about ten minutes. Their surfaces will be frozen, now they won't lump together when you add them to a zip-lock bag or container.

You can do this same process with fruit. You need to remove any cores and pits. But you do not need to blanch them before freezing.

➢ **Mark The Dates**: If the container does not have an expiration date, use a sharpie marker to add on the date it was bought or cooked.

➢ **Leftovers**: Waste not, Want not. We will go over leftovers in more detail later. However, it is good to note that burritos, casseroles, soups/stews, and stir-fries all freeze well. And they retain most of their flavor when you rewarm them. Almost anything can be converted into one of these things for meals made from leftovers.

➢ **Make Breakfast In Bulk**: Busy mornings? Don't rush to the fast food line. Find a day to make protein rich pancakes, biscuits, and waffles. Avoid enriched white flour. It doesn't offer the protein or nutritional value of wheat flour or ground oats. These can be added to zip bags and frozen for a quick warmup in the mornings.

Invest in an emulsifier and make green smoothies for breakfast.

➤ **Leftovers For Lunch**: A thermos is a wonderful thing. You can heat up leftovers and pack it in the thermos. You or your child now has a warm meal come lunchtime.

➤ **Smoothies**: Fruit and some ice, blended for about 30 seconds. If you want it creamy, add some milk or soy milk. When you get adventurous, you can check recipes that add in vegetables.

It is a cold, healthy treat that only takes a minute to make. It is far cheaper than ice cream or Starbucks, with none of the extra sugar.

➤ **Use Your Freezer:** You can make anything you see in the freezer aisle from scratch. Freeze them into meal and single serving sizes. Your version will have less sodium and artificial preservatives.

➤ **Zipbags:** Freeze rice dishes in zip bags with the air carefully displaced. They take up less room in the freezer than tupperware. Some of the higher quality bags can even be used to store soup and stew the same way! Make sure they are frozen before stacking other things on them.

➤ **Herbs:** Too many fresh herbs? Make soup stock and freeze it in ice trays. Transfer them into zip bags or tupperware dishes. Now you just take out a few to flavor your dishes.

> **Make Specialty Coffee At Home**: With far less sugar and fat too. For example: combine coffee, soy milk, ice, fresh mint (or a drop of imitation mint flavor), and a spoonful of unsweetened cocoa powder. Mix or blend well for your own mint mocha.

> **Baby Food:** Baby food is unspiced regular food finely pureed in a food processor. Check out sites maintained by a pediatrician or child nutritionist for preservative free recipes and proper storage.

Leftovers

There are hundreds of thousands of recipes dedicated to using leftovers to create a new dish. This greatly reduces food waste, and it stretches your budget for an extra meal. You can find entire books dedicated to the practice in libraries and online resources. Here are a few ideas to get you started:

> **Soup Stock**: You can make soup stock by boiling the bones left over from dinner before discarding them. It is generally healthier than store bought broth. There are no extra preservatives, and you control the salt content (if any). Any bones, fish, shrimp shells, and veggies will work. Try making your own chicken and vegetable stock.

> **Meats**: Just about any extra meat can be added to soup, brown rice, or beans to create a whole new meal.

> **Lean Chicken Salad**: Remove the skin and bones. Put meat and a tablespoon of Italian dressing into food processor. Mix in diced desired veggies, like onions or bell pepper. Its now ready for a whole wheat sandwich or a salad.

> **French Toast**: If your bread goes stale, you can still make one more meal out of them. Mix up egg whites and low fat or soy

milk. Soak the hardened bread in the mixture, then cook them in a pan or skillet. Top with fruit and nuts instead of sugar and syrup. These are high in protein and some vital minerals when you use whole grain breads. However, they are also high in calories and some fats. Be mindful of portion sizes.

➢ **Old Vegetables** can be frozen for another day. They can also be added into soups, casseroles, and rice dishes.

➢ **Vegetable Stir-Fry**: Too many side dishes? Cook leftover veggies in a pan with a tablespoon of sunflower or olive oil. Serve with brown rice.

➢ **Tortillas**: Roll leftover beans and sliced lean meat into a whole grain tortilla for a quick and easy portable lunch. The protein and fiber is better for you than that value menu burger. Add in diced onions, lettuce and tomatoes for extra depth.

Don't forget to check out the library and the internet for a host of free recipes. **Each extra meal you salvage from your leftovers is money saved.**

Gardening

Gardening is a great way to add in healthy, organic produce to your diet. It is also the only way to completely know what you are putting into your body. You control the soil used. You control whether or not fertilizer or pesticides are used, and what kind.

You do not need a large space to begin gardening. Even a sunny spot by the window can produce fresh herbs and a few tomatoes. Here are few unconventional ideas to consider.

➢ **Landscape Gardening**: Use your normal landscaping for edible plants. Fruit and/or nut bearing trees provide shade and décor. Edible flowers are added into the flower beds. Flowering berry bushes can act as hedges for the yard.

➢ **Vertical Gardening**: This is great for small and medium sized yards. The plants are rooted in the ground but then are coaxed into growing upwards onto trellises or nets. This greatly expands the area space by letting your melons, squash, and other produce grow in midair.

➢ **Container Gardening**: This is ideal for small spaces or urban living. As the name implies, your fruit trees, berry bushes, and vegetables are all grown in containers. It can be anything from a teacup to a thirty gallon ceramic bowl on wheels. This gives you full control over your garden. You can move it to shelter in bad weather. You can move the plants closer to water or shade. You can even have a garden indoors or on your patio/balcony.

➢ **Aquaponic Garden**: This Garden is more advanced, and it takes up a lot of room. It forms a symbiotic relationship between your garden and edible fish. It also has a large initial cost, with long term savings and benefits. Once it is set up, the fish provide fertilizer, and the plants provide oxygenated water, no filters or motors necessary.

There are 'pet' versions as well. You grow herbs over a specially built tank for pet fish. These mini-gardens are even sold on Amazon and Ebay. It is a way to become acquainted with the process before going 'all in' with a full sized model.

➢ **Community Gardens**: The recent rise in health awareness has encouraged the growth of community gardens. You sign up with your town hall, and you get a plot of land to take care of. Depending on your location, the rules and possible fees will vary.

Thrifty Tip: Some areas offers tax deductions for gardening and bee keeping. San Francisco's *Urban Agriculture Incentive Zones Act* did just that for urban and community farm owners in 2014. Check with your State Agricultural Department for local laws and incentives.

A garden can fit right into your lifestyle, whether it is landscaping or a few containers for salad greens.

Milk and Meat

Food animals require space, food, and care. However, if you have the space and the discipline, keeping a milk goat or some egg laying hens can provide for your protein needs.

Preferably, you can cut the meat altogether. However, raising your own animals guarantee they receive no growth hormones or unnecessary antibiotics. Also, a butcher will custom cut and seal the portions for you.

If raising your own meat animal is not for you, you can also buy them directly from the farm (you can even split the cost with 1-2 other families). The animal will be delivered to the butcher, and each share is custom cut to each family's needs. While it is a steep up-front price, you save a great deal on the price per pound. Especially when you account for ribs, fresh tongue and liver, and choice cut meats.

The meat needs to be vacuum sealed to get the best value. This way, it will last up to a year in the freezer.

There are many more ways to stretch your budget outside of the grocery store. However, these tips should be a handy way to get started.

Chapter 6: Social Strategies

Food brings people together on many different levels
– Giada de Laurentiis

We are social creatures. We need to touch base with other human beings, some more frequently than others. This need to connect with other humans has endured since prehistoric times. It was very practical, after all. Groups protected and supported each other. Groups could bring in larger game and harvests. Groups shared their bounty in good times and bad.

This connection is so ingrained that we have designed ways to stay connected all the time. While group hunting and gathering is a rarity, our gatherings still almost always involve food.

We can make it through these social events without tearing apart our budget. In fact, we can even use our social networks to save money on our monthly groceries.

Parties / Events

Interactions often revolve around food. Birthday parties, holidays and first dates are just a few examples. When we raise a family, we find ourselves host to a flurry of events. Sleepovers, post-recital celebrations, school events, sports... the commitments grow faster than the children at times.

While each of these events is important, they are also a budget trap for the hostess. Also, there are always surprise events, extra guests, and other curveballs to adapt to.

A social function does not need to break the bank. With a little planning, you can cut these extra costs significantly.

> ➢ **Be Mindful at Potlucks:** Potlucks and group picnics can be a great way to stretch a budget. You bring a dish to share, and you can eat a variety of foods that other guests bring.

However, many of these foods are not healthy, like the sodium saturated hot dogs. It is easy to consume *over a thousand* calories in a single meal. If you do attend such an event, be mindful of what goes on your plate.

➢ **Make Your Appetizer Trays:** Bags of baby carrots, broccoli, and other veggies are cheaper individually than in party trays. The same goes for buying grapes, apples, strawberries, and pineapple. Slice as needed, and create your own trays.

➢ **Use Your Food Processor:** Make your own fresh, low sodium salsa, bean dip, and hummus. Recipes can be found online.

➢ **Make Your Own Tortilla Chips:** Slice tortillas with a sharp knife or pizza cutter. Then bake in oven for 10 minutes at 425 degrees. Cooking times may vary for desired crispness.

➢ **Bake Your Own Cakes:** Does it have to be a huge birthday sheet cake? Cake is a common tradition on the big day, so it might be difficult to decide on a different main dessert. Even if the cake isn't healthy, it can be *healthier*. You could use a different flour. You could make small cupcakes for portion control. Also look up "low cost diabetic desserts' to find out lots of alternative sugar-free treats. Nondairy whip instead of butter cream, applesauce instead of sugar...You might even forgo a cake altogether. How about about colorful parfaits or rainbow gelatin molds?

➢ **Use Flavoring Additives Instead Of Syrups:** A few drops go a LONG way. Small bottles are found in the baking aisle, and they pack a lot of flavor. They come in a host of flavors from vanilla to mint. You can flavor coffees, ginger ale, or crushed ice very inexpensively. Better yet, it does not have the sugar or extra calories of flavor syrups.

➤ **Make Your Own Gourmet Ice Cream:** It only takes two Ziploc bags and rock salt. Instructions and recipes are abundant online. Use nuts, berries, fruit, or imitation flavoring to create your own signature flavor.

➤ **Make It A Potluck:** At your next event, provide the main dish, a drink, and the main dessert. Have the guests bring their favorite side dishes, casseroles, and appetizers. This is especially helpful when you are accounting for a host of dietary restrictions. Be mindful of the portions that go on your plate, however.

➤ **Save On The Decorations:** Make your first stop a 99 cent store or Dollar tree. You can find matching tablecloths, plates, napkins and utensils for very cheap. You may even find center pieces, Mylar balloons, and party hats. They come in a wide variety of colors and licensed characters.

➤ **Invest In A Large Rolling Cooler:** Stock it with water, juice, and healthy finger foods for big events. If you have treats on hand, you are less likely to buy those over-priced concession foods or stop for fast food on the way home.

➤ **Redefine 'Going Out':** A date night or family outing does not need to involve a restaurant. Save those for extra special occasions.

Instead, pack a meal and see what the community has to offer. Find an outdoor movie. Check the event calendars for free plays, hikes, and festivals. Hunt out 'hidden treasures' around your area. Put the phones on silent and enjoy time together by a park lake.

Social Media

Modern technology makes it easier for people to connect with one another. More importantly, it allows us to find deals and opportunities more effectively.

> **Check Social Media Sites For Buy/Swap/Sell Groups:** You can find anything from baby clothes to nearly new furniture. On rare occasion, you will even find people giving away extra produce or eggs. You can also unload extra clutter when you need a few dollars.

> **Seek Out Local Bee Keepers, Farmers, Butchers And Others:** Follow or bookmark their websites or social media pages. Check once a week or so for updates on cheap or free fresh goods.

> **Create Bookoo And Craigslist Accounts:** You can create ISO's (In Search Of) posts to find practically anything. They also have "Free" and "Barter" zones where you could find free surplus nuts, berries, and produce. Remember to always meet at safe, public places. Practice safe meeting habits.

> **Find Coupon Groups on Facebook:** Read up on great sales and trade Sunday paper coupons with one another.

> **Thrifty Tip**: Online printouts of manufacturer's coupons usually have a limit of two copies per computer. Arrange coupon swaps to get extras you need.

Bartering / Skill Swaps

Bartering is an age old tradition. Long before printed currency, we traded our skills and extra supplies for the things we needed.

> **It Is All About *Value*:** Some people are intimidated by bartering because there is no distinct price tag. They would

rather just pay a price and be done. Bartering is about making the trade mutually beneficial to both sides. It does not need to be financially equal if both sides are happy.

➢ **Bumper Crop:** Did you grow more produce than you can use? Check around with friends and social media groups. Someone might be willing to trade babysitting services, lend out a prom dress, or trade a few jars of blackberry jelly for them. Be sure to outline exactly what you hope to gain in your query.

➢ **Skills Trade Well:** Skills are an infinite resource. You can repeat it indefinitely. You do something for the other person, and you receive something in return. It also relieves a financial burden from you both. They get a needed skill, and you get a product or some items you need.

Would someone do all your canning for you in exchange for a custom handmade rag doll? Can you barter your math tutoring skills for fresh honey and homemade cheese? Can you bead a necklace to match their daughter's homecoming dress?

Group Efforts

Cooking can feel tedious. Especially if you live a very busy lifestyle. If you have access to a large kitchen, consider a cooking meet-up.

Everyone is assigned a fair share of the ingredient list for meals. They each buy, barter, or produce their share on meet day. Everyone then works together to make meals and socialize.

When everything is done, everyone gets their fair share. They take their goods home and freeze them. Now all they need to do is rewarm the food for meals as needed for the rest of the week.

As you can see, we can avoid breaking our budget with a little planning. In fact, with patience we can even stretch our budgets.

Of course, there are times when budgeting and planning is not enough. We need extra funds to make it through. In the next chapter, we will expand into ways to increase our available funds.

Chapter 7: Increase Income

While most people are shrinking their dreams constantly to fit within their income circle, 2% of the population are finding ways to increase their income to fit their dreams' circle. – ***Dani Johnson***

Sometimes budgets, coupons, and sales are not enough. There are no good sales for the week. The free sites will be dry. Bartering is not getting us everything we need. This is why we need extra income to boost our budget.

We can not always take on extra hours at work. We won't receive bonuses or pay raises on demand. Some of us out there *cannot* go to work for various reasons.

There is now a vast world of methods we can use to attain extra funds. None of them are guaranteed to bring in huge sums. Many of them take time to develop. However, every little bit helps. If you made $10 from five things, you just made $50. If you do exceptionally well in one thing, you could make hundreds or more in extra funds.

Important Notes:

1. *These are not a paycheck.* Unlike a job, these techniques do not guarantee income. Do not put them in the main budget before they have been earned. Instead, make them 'discretionary' funds for debt payment, events, and extra groceries.

2. *It's still taxable.* You have to declare almost all forms of income on your taxes. In some places, you even need to declare gift cards and lottery winnings. In most cases, these random sources will fall under "other income." When in doubt, check with a tax professional.

3. *Invest in a ledger.* Even if it is just a notebook with a pocket for receipts. This will help you keep track of what works best

for bringing money in. It will also be a HUGE help come tax time.

4. *Consider signing up for a Square or PayPal account.* These services allow you to take credit/debit cards anywhere with wifi access, and they keep track of your sales for you. There are no monthly fees, and the transaction fees are reasonable. You do not need a reader compatible devise (though you keep more money per transaction if you use it). You can enter the transactions manually, if needed.

Income Ideas:

➢ **Garage Sale**: A garage sale lets you clean out your clutter, and it provides quick cash. Make sure to price tag everything. It is not unusual to make $150 to $300 or more in a weekend selling off clutter and big ticket items.

➢ **Consignment Shops**: Some shops are set up to allow you to rent space to sell your extra stuff. Others buy the item off you on the spot. Stick with gently used objects. Make sure they are clean and wrinkle free. Make sure toys and games are not missing pieces.

➢ **Online Consignment**: Like physical shops, an online consignment shop either buys the object from you or gives you 'space' to sell it yourself. You do need to send your items in to be inspected and graded.

Swap.com is a consignment shop where you can trade or sell your gently used clothes, books, child decor, and more. As of 2016, they also took nearly new books and DVDs up to PG13. They also recently expanded into woman's clothing.

Thredup.com, on the other hand, is selective about the clothes they take. However, they pay you on the spot.

➤ **EBay/Amazon**: Online market websites allow you to sell to them outright, or you can post an ad in their marketplace. You can sell new or used items. You can even sell vehicles, collectables, and vintage items. If you are hosting an event, you can post the tickets on EBay if you meet their criteria.

There is usually a holding period on your first earnings. In general this freeze lasts from two to four weeks. This is to protect the consumer's from 'fly by night' scams. Once trust has been established, you can get to your earnings almost immediately.

➤ **ETSY**: If you are skilled with handmade products or vintage items, you can sell your goods on ETSY. You can even sell pdf's of your own crafting instructions, crafting components, and raw supplies. People even sell pine needles and boxes of empty toilet paper rolls for class projects.

➤ **Rent Out Your Stuff**: Do you use your shampooer only once a month or so? Is the PS3 collecting dust? Why not let them make money for you between uses? You can rent out practically anything on sites like Zilok. If you make $20 a week renting out a spare 3DS system, it would mean up to $80 in a month. Note: Always take a deposit in case something happens. The deposit should cover full replacement in the event of loss, theft, or breakage.

➤ **Rent a Room**: Places like airBnB help you rent out that spare room or couch to travelers. Make sure to treat your valuables responsibly. Describe the space and any extras (like breakfast included) accurately.

➤ **Sitter**. There is always someone that needs a child, plant, pet, or house watched over. If you enjoy caring for others, this could be a way to make some extra cash. Make sure your rates ensure a profit after expenses (gas, food for kids, etc). Keep in mind that some states require you to have a license before you advertise outside of friends and family.

➢ **Driver**: Sites like Lyft.com and Uber are hiring independent drivers. You have to have your own vehicle, insurance, and keep gas money on hand. However, you also get to dictate your driving hours and range. They get a cut of every ride they send your way.

➢ **Tutoring:** Are you particularly good at an academic subject? You could make $30+ an hour tutoring students. The more vital (SAT's) and complex (advanced chemistry) the subject, the more you can charge.

➢ **Teach a Skill**: There are many people who make extra funds by teaching others. You can do a set fee or 'by donation' rate. The skills you can teach are infinite: painting, dancing, basic crochet, using Pinterest... even how to send an email or download a kindle book. If you are particularly tech savvy, you could even set up online classes on sites like Udemy and Skillshare.

➢ **Freelance**: You can freelance almost any skill online these days. You can make money off a hobby, a talent, or formal education. You can find relatively easy entry-level jobs on sites like Freelance.com and Upwork. Variety sites like Fiverr allow freelancers to do fun and goofy things for a quick Five bucks. For example, one person sings Happy Birthday in a Scottish accent, and sends the recipient the video file.

➢ **Personal Assistant/Virtual Assistant**: You can charge a flat fee or an hourly rate to help others with simple, time-consuming tasks. It could be anything from picking up their dry cleaning to posting blogs on their social media. You might even use your new shopping skills to take care of their grocery trips.

➤ **Sell to Local Shops and Restaurants**: Do you have a surplus of fresh nuts or dried herbs? Do you make an amazing sugar free, whole grain cobbler? See if a local store or restaurant would like to buy from you. Make sure you do not need a license or nutritional labels first. You'll make a better impression if you are in compliance with local laws. The Clerk of court office can point you in the right direction regarding local laws.

➤ **Gift Cards**: If you spend a lot of time doing internet searches and watching videos, you can convert that idle time into gift cards. Rewards programs like Bing and Swagbucks reward you with points when you participate. You then turn these points into gift cards.

If you do not like the available cards, you can sell, gift, or barter the more popular ones for things you need. For example, a New Mexico mother collects Starbucks and Movie gift cards. Then she trades them off for kids' clothes and video games on a FaceBook swap site. These games are quietly stashed away for birthdays and holidays.

➤ **Blogging/Affiliate Marketing**: As a word of warning: this process rarely creates a substantial income in the first six months. You will need to build a dedicated reader base of people likely to buy things you suggest. If sharing your experiences and knowledge is a passion, you can sell ad space and guest post privileges. You can link your blogs to affiliate products. There are a host of ways to monetize your blog.

There are hundreds of other ways to make extra money online. Test the waters with a few of these. Afterward, focus on building up one or two that you enjoy doing the most.

Conclusion

You can eat very healthy on a budget. It just takes extra planning. It can be as simple as learning a few recipes or being mindful of what goes in the cart. You can use circulars to find the best sales. You can plan meals ahead of time.

You now have the resources to find healthy, local foods. You even have ways to increase your income when things are getting tight.

Everything covered in this book lays the foundation. I hope you will use these tools and strategies to live a healthier and happier life.

Appendix 1: Menu Planner

You can print this out or create one of your own. Chapter 1 covers how to make the best use of a plan.

Breakfast:

_____

_____

Lunch:

_____

_____

Dinner:

_____

_____

Grocery List:

_____	_____
_____	_____
_____	_____
_____	_____

Appendix 2: Simple Budget

Date: _____

Grocery Budget For Month: _____

    Week 1: _____   Week 2: _____

    Week 3: _____   Week 4: _____

    Events to Plan For:

_____

_____

    Top Staples Needed:

_____   _____

_____   _____

_____   _____

_____   _____

_____   _____

_____   _____

References

Economides, Steve, and Annette Economides. *Cut Your Grocery Bill in Half with America's Cheapest Family: Includes so Many Innovative Strategies You Won't Have to Cut Coupons*. Nashville, TN: Thomas Nelson, 2010. Print.

Extraordinary Uses for Ordinary Things: 2,317 Ingenious Uses for Vinegar, Salt, Coffee Grounds, String, Pantyhose, Mayonnaise, Clothespins, Aspirin, and More than 200 Other Common Household Items. N.p.: Reader's Digest, n.d. Print.

"How to Save Money on Groceries: Tips for Frugal Shoppers."*How to Save Money on Groceries: Tips for Frugal Shoppers*. N.p., n.d. Web. 04 May 2016. <http://www.alwaysfrugal.com/groceries.html>.

"Zen Habits: 50 Tips for Grocery Shopping."*Zen Habits RSS*. N.p., n.d. Web. 04 May 2016. <http://zenhabits.net/50-tips-for-grocery-shopping/>.

About The Author

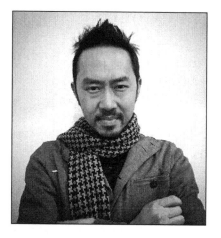

Dr. Duc Vuong

Dr. Duc Vuong is an internationally renowned bariatric surgeon, who is the world's leading expert in education for the bariatric patient.

His intensive educational system has garnered attention from multiple institutions and medical societies. His passion in life is to fill the shortage of educational resources between patients and weight loss surgeons.

Although trained in Western medicine, he blends traditional Eastern teachings with the latest in science and technology. Dr. Vuong was featured in TLC's hit show, 900 Pound Man: Race Against Time, and is currently working on his own weekly television show.

Visit Dr. Duc Vuong on

www.UltimateGastricSleeve.com

to learn more.

Other Books by Dr. Duc Vuong

...available on Amazon.com

Meditate to Lose Weight: A Guide For A Slimmer Healthier You

Healthy Green Smoothies: 50 Easy Recipes That Will Change Your Life

Big-Ass Salads: 31 Easy Recipes For Your Healthy Month

Weight Loss Surgery Success: Dr. V's A-Z Steps For Losing Weight And Gaining Enlightenment

The Ultimate Gastric Sleeve Success: A Practical Patient Guide

Lap-Band Struggles: Revisit. Rethink. Revise.

Leave Me a Review!

If you enjoyed this book or found it useful, please take a moment to leave a review on Amazon. I'm always interested in learning what you like, think and want. I read all the reviews personally.

Thank you for your support!

50473412R00035

Made in the USA
Middletown, DE
31 October 2017